GETTING RIPPED

MICHAEL SMYTH

ISBN-13: 978-1523239252
ISBN-10: 1523239255

THE REAL SECRET TO GAIN MUSCLE AND GET RIPPED IN JUST 12 WEEKS

CONTENTS

INTRODUCTION

There are many supplement companies doing transformation challenges around the country today. Many offer incredible prizes like new sports cars, cash, appearances in films, jobs and many other things. I learned first-hand about these challenges about ten years ago when I too was motivated to do my first challenge. First prize was about a quarter of a million dollars in cash and prizes. I thought to myself "This could be a game changer for me." I knew that I could get into incredible shape and come away with some amazing cash and prizes! I decided to put everything I had into it. I read up on supplements, I checked out the best diet advice, I read about which exercises and routines were best to use. I bought hundreds of dollars in special supplements and hundreds more in special foods, I followed their advice and put a huge effort into it. I really wanted to win. I asked myself..."Am I really willing to do what it will take to be a winner in this?" and my answer was yes. I would give an "all out" effort.

Here is where the problem came into play...You see it wasn't that I didn't try hard enough. I was not lazy by any stretch of the imagination. I would get up at four a.m. to be at the gym by five just to ride the bike for an hour. I did afternoon work outs... I put my heart into it....

In the end... I really was in much better shape than I had been in for a long time. But I wasn't close to being where I needed to be to win. When it was all said and done, I completed the 12 week challenge 3 times. I learned that most of the advice I had received about diet, supplements, cardio and workouts was not taking me where I needed to go. It was good, solid advice for workouts in general, but not for winning a contest. It took me three times but I finally figured it out. I got the revelation about what it really takes to win.... And I share it here.

But first... Let me tell you a little about by Transformation Contest experiences....

1
MY FIRST TWO
"TRANSFORMATIONS"

Going in...

I am going to tell you about my experiences and I am going to be real with you. If you are going to do this transformation thing, you should know in advance that it will be one of the most wonderful experiences of your life. But you also have to know the whole story. What it really takes to get there and be a contender. In my opinion, it's more important to know this than it is to hear about another type of sit-up and how to do it, or to read about new twists on old exercises. (That stuff is important too. We have to know what we're doing so we are not spinning our wheels and wasting time.)

When I first read about the transformation challenge that I ended up doing, I was stoked! I knew I needed something to shake me out of my complacency to being out of shape and I believed that this contest thing could do it. The company that was conducting it was reputable and their products were awesome so there wasn't anything really standing in my way.

At the time, I weighed 248 lbs. Ouch! It hurts just writing it. My optimum weight is about 200 lbs. I know that the charts say for my height I should be 185 lbs., but I would be emaciated at that weight.

I had never done something this challenging before. To go from being 50 lbs. overweight and being completely out of shape, to being athletic and ripped seemed like a fantasy to me quite frankly and then, to make matters even more unbelievable, to do it in only 12 weeks! But I had seen pictures of many who had done it and I got past my initial doubts. I decided wholeheartedly to do it and not hold back. I would do it to win, and I would put in the effort, whatever that was, to make it happen. I would commit.

I had no idea what kind of effort it would take because I had never done it before. I didn't know what kind of sacrifices would be required or adjustments to my life that would have to be made. I didn't know the oppositions I would face or where they would come from. I just knew that the "prize" or the goal would be worth the effort.

Getting My "Team" On Board

Because I knew that this was going to take a commitment of both time and money, I talked to my wife about it to get her approval and commitment to help me. I know that I do not need anyone's approval to get into shape. I know that. But it is always better to include your spouse or the person closest to you so that you have someone who knows what you are doing and someone willing to be an helper in the process. I knew that the 12 week process would require a commitment from both of us so that I could be free to give it all I had.

Money was also a factor in getting my wife in agreement. I was going to spend several hundreds of dollars on supplements and special foods. I did not have money set aside for this so it would have to come out of our regular budget. Thankfully, my wife could see what a great gift it would be to the family for me to be healthy and in shape. She was not moved by the prizes but by the health reasons. She agreed it was something that would benefit our family.

Again, I could have just spent the money and bought what I needed, but I am trying to use this little segment to also teach a reality in doing this. It is always better to do this from a place of everyone being on the same page. Doing the competition or transformation from an atmosphere of cooperation and encouragement is so much more conducive to success than waking up every day to a battle and trying to be successful in the middle of that battle. I really hope you take this to heart.

Again, time and other things would play a factor, because for 12 weeks my wife would have to understand that there were going to be restaurants where I would not eat. If we had to go, I would take my own food with me. (Please don't be embarrassed) Also many times she would have to go to places by herself because I had workouts scheduled. To an outsider, it may sound selfish but sacrifice is needed for success. It was 12 weeks where things would be different. We could get back to normal afterwards.

Research and Preparation

I read everything that I could find on people making these "transformations." I read many, many things from the companies that were conducting them. I could find precious little from the people who had actually done them and what they might have learned in the process. I read article after article about the best workouts, nutrition, fat loss, supplements and how to use them, health concerns, the most effective cardio and other related factors.

I found out what times were going to be best for me to get in my workouts and cardio sessions so that they could flow seamlessly into my normal life as much as possible.

I looked at which foods would be the cheapest and easiest to have on hand for my goals. I covered all the bases as much as I could.

I picked a start date and I ordered all of the product that I would need in advance. I chose meal replacement packets that I could mix with water that were about 300 calories each. I chose Creatine to promote muscle growth (from what I had read) I chose glutamine to preserve muscle mass and protect my gains. I also ordered a handful of meal replacement bars just in case. My wife stocked up on lean beef, turkey, chicken and tuna. She also stocked the pantry with complex carbs like oatmeal and sweet potatoes and brown rice. Many other foods that were said to help were also purchased.

Getting Ready to do Pictures

I spent all of that time telling you about how important it is to get people in your corner as you do your challenge and now I will show you why. You see, when I found out about this challenge I got excited about it and decided to share this transformation challenge thing with a good friend who had also let himself get out of shape. He got excited as well! At the time, we talked about doing workouts together and encouraging each other etc., and taking each other's before and after photos and all that. He really wanted to do it too.

When I hadn't heard from him in several weeks, I decided to call him a week prior to doing the challenge to figure out when we could get together to do the pictures, he said that yes, he was still very excited to be doing the challenge but found someone else to do it with. A guy at the gym was a competitive bodybuilder and they were going to do the workouts together and photos and all that. But thanks anyway...

It was a very discouraging moment for me. I didn't react. I just said "That's great. I hope you do very well." And then found a reason to get off the phone. I could have spent more time feeling sorry for myself... I am the one who told him about this, and all that... But I was very happy at that time that my wife was totally on board and she became my encourager throughout the process and she also did my pictures for me. In hind-sight it was probably for the best.

The Pictures

The day we did the pictures was an experience. I was a bit embarrassed to let my stomach relax in front of her. Lol! I waited until late in the evening and then asked her to take them. I realized afterwards that if you are 50 lbs. overweight, you don't have to try to look overweight. We did about 20 – 30 pictures from various angles all in line with what the contest pictures had shown from others who were chosen in the competition literature. The "after" pictures require a lot more attention.

The Workout

My workouts were serious and I was all business. (Although I enjoyed them) I am not going to go into a lot of detail on this end because I don't recommend what I was doing at this point. But I Basically was doing an hour to an hour and a half workout every day except Sunday, splitting my workouts so as to give my muscle groups time to recover. i.e. biceps and back one day, and triceps and chest the next... or something similar.

The weight I was using at first was very light. I was starting out with twenty lb. dumbbells for curls for example. I put effort into it though and always felt that I had done a real workout. The first time I did not go real heavy because of advice I had read in a fitness magazine, and the second time I did go real heavy because of what I had read in a fitness magazine. Go figure...

I covered all of the muscle groups, working each group with proper form etc.. For the most part, the actual weights workout I did was pretty good I would say. It was almost on the mark and I will share that later. If you are following a laid out workout from a reputable trainer or expert, you are probably going to be in the ballpark. As long as at the end of the workout, you can feel it, you are making strides.

The Cardio

This is one area where taking the expert advice was a mistake. (Actually, there were several factors that together created the problem) I had read that high-intensity, interval cardio workouts were the absolute best for a cardio workout. The guy giving the advice was ripped and that always plays a part in credibility. However, we have to remember that he may have already been ripped, and probably was. Its not like he was overweight a year ago and these workouts were what got him to where he is.

But the premise is sound though. So I was doing two, twenty minute cardio sessions on the stair-stepper or the exercise bike about five days a week. In addition to regular workouts excluding leg days. I would do a two minute warmup and then launch into a one minute normal, thirty second intense and then repeat throughout with a two minute cool down. I could feel it. I really did help. I know it did. But to win I found that you need more.

In all the workout and cardio information I had been reading, the conventional wisdom was that less cardio, more focus on building muscle was the key to getting ripped. It sounds good because we know that muscle burns fat even when you are at rest. The thing that they and we fail to grasp is that we only have the twelve weeks and that is not the way to do it if you have no time. You have to have both in the right amounts to achieve the right results.

My first day on the stair stepper I forced myself to do six minutes because one of the trainers at the gym was watching me. I felt like I was going to die at the end of six minutes. But at the end of the week I was doing fifteen and by the end of the second week I was doing my twenty minute cardio sessions and really putting myself into it. On my second go around (competition) I increased cardio almost double. It helped to give me even better results on the second try.

I stuck mainly on the bike and stair-stepper, although I did use the treadmill many times also to kind of break things up. Again, I was doing ok. I did end up getting into great shape and being very strong but I was not in contest winning shape by any stretch of the imagination.

My Calorie Intake

This was one area that I really blew it. I followed the advice in the magazines very closely on this one. I guess I did because it made no logical sense to me that I should consume 3,500 calories to fuel my workouts and lose fat, so I figured that this had to be one of the important "missing ingredients" that most people don't get. As I told you, my wife bought all the right foods and I tried my best to eat that much food as much as I could.

I was eating according to what all the pros and experts were saying I should do. I split my meals up into six meals throughout the day. I had also read that you should have a "cheat day" if you want to be successful. It gives you a psychological boost that allows you to think you are not being deprived and throws your metabolism a "curve ball" that it has to adjust to. (At least that was how it was explained to me) The cheat day is one concept you have to pay close attention to in a contest like these 12 - week things. You can derail your whole effort by not doing that right.

Anyway... I enjoyed my cheat days and it was nice to eat other foods on those days.

My Results

On the very first contest, I lost about forty lbs. and came out of it in great shape. My waist measurement went from forty-eight inches down to thirty- three. I felt wonderful. My clothes fit me so well I felt like a million bucks even if I would put on rags. It's funny how that works like that. I was strong at the end of these twelve weeks. I could bench 300 for two reps. I could do cardio for an hour if I wanted to. I was doing curls with 40 or 45 lib. Dumbbells. I had energy like crazy. My mental state was incredible. I felt great! I think that win or lose, doing something like this makes you come out a winner just in all these other facets. But....

How did I do contest-wise? That's what we're talking about right? The truth was that I was not close to being ripped. I still had my body fat at about twelve percent. It was just low enough that I could see the outline of my abs, but there was no real definition.

I had realized at about ten weeks that I couldn't possibly get where I needed to be in only two more weeks. It was discouraging but I rode it out by continuing to follow their advice just in case there was some miracle that happened somehow at the last minute. I gave it all I had until the very last day. Then I did the after pictures but I knew I was not even close. I could compare my results with the photos of others and began to think "How in the world did they get those results doing the same thing that I did?"

Please bare with me as I share my journey with you... I am telling you this for a reason. I am expecting you to believe what I am about to tell you and the reason you can believe me is because you have heard about my successes and failures. Everything I will tell you I learned first-hand. These things are not just good ideas I read somewhere in a book. This is tried and true my friend. You can trust I'm steering you in the right direction.

On my second contest try, I made some serious changes and I did much, much better. But in the end it still was not what it needed to be. My third attempt was where I threw conventional wisdom out the window and did what I thought made the most sense. And that attempt got me ripped.

And that is the program I will now share with you.

2
PREPARATION
START AT THE BEGINNING

Getting Your Mind Right

This first thing you have to come to grips with if you are going to do this in twelve weeks is that this is what your life is going to be about for that twelve week period. Of course I'm not talking about quitting your job or ignoring your family, but rather that there will really be no free time to speak of. You have to decide if you are willing to sacrifice your free time. I mention it because it isn't really an option here. I have told you that I learned what it takes and this really is part of it. Are you willing to sacrifice sleep to get that workout in? Will you do your hour of cardio even when you don't feel like it. Decide going in and it will make it much easier when the temptations come to miss a workout. If you have already made up your mind, you can just move ahead .

What Image do You Have of Yourself?

Part of getting your mind right is having an idea of what you want your body to look like. It is a target goal of sorts. You should get online or go through some magazines and find several good photos that inspire you and that you would be happy to look like.

You can't use negative reinforcement because it does not work. It pulls you the wrong way. I know it may seem like if you would see a picture of someone who is overweight, maybe even yourself, it would motivate you to change. That just is not the case. It becomes a depressive thing. You are constantly reminded you are fat (or overweight) and it becomes just another obstacle to overcome.

Find a goal picture and look at it several times a day and just tell yourself, either silently or out loud "This is me." "This is how I look." I don't want to get into quantum physics, but there is scientific evidence that we can literally change things physically by speaking to a situation. If you doubt this, look online or on You tube for experiments with sounds or the effects of words on crystals, water, plants etc.. This is one reason that you should do this. The other reason is because of good old fashioned positive reinforcement.

Keep your mind and thoughts going in the same direction as your goals. I found this to be very important because as you pursue something like this, your focus and commitment is very crucial. Many times others around your life will not be supportive of your goal or quest on an ongoing basis so you have to be your own best "cheer leader."

Get Ready For Opposition

Which brings us to this point. There will be people around you who just don't get it. Oh when you first start they will say "That's great!" but a week in, they will be giving you brownies. People that wouldn't make something for you ever will be baking their little hearts out. "What do you mean you can't eat this?! I made this specially for you! Just one...ok?" They won't come out and say "I'm trying to sabotage you." But unconsciously they are doing exactly that. You will suddenly find that you are expected to go out for dinner for some reason and you are expected to eat "normal." You have to plan for stuff like this and think ahead. Have an idea of what you would eat if you had to go to a restaurant.

It's not just about food either. Have an idea of how you will make up workouts you miss without burning yourself out. What I have found is that it is almost impossible to keep your schedule completely on schedule if you have any other commitments going on in your life. Someone in your life may know that you need to be at the gym from four thirty until six, but they will schedule something else at five. And then be miffed that you wouldn't blow off your workout "just this once." I know it sounds funny, but this is all stuff that I have had to deal with and others I know have dealt with the same thing. You just have to be aware so that you can have a plan in place to handle it and not be discouraged by the perceived lack of support.

You may be fine in these areas and if so...great. But if not at least you will have had a heads up so that you can stay focused on the goal and not get dragged down.

Get Your Food and Supplements Ready

One of the thing that set me back the first couple times that I did this was not being completely prepared for my meals. It is very hard to eat clean if you have not already made that provision for yourself. When ten o'clock comes and it's time to eat (or take in calories) if you are having to scavenge for food, chances are it will not be something healthy from your approved list.

I went through this many times. I would go somewhere knowing that I had plenty of time to make it to a store or back home for my meal and something would happen to mess up my schedule. If the only thing available is a snack machine, even the healthiest choice is probably still junk. I began carrying small protein bars everywhere I went for this reason. If it came down to it, I could eat the protein bar. Sometimes, several times actually I have had to eat them for several meals in a day because things just worked out that way.

One thing to also keep in mind is that just because the guy on the wrapper is ripped, doesn't mean the product is good for you or will help you with your goals. Be aware of the break-down of calories, and how it fits into your game plan. We will cover that later.

Also keep in mind that you may have to make some meals in advance the day or night before and store them in some kind of air tight container. This way your meals will be ready so that you can stay on schedule. You should buy some extra, inexpensive containers and have them hidden and ready to use when the need arises. There is sometimes a possibility that someone may use your containers unless you mark them somehow so that everyone knows they are spoken for. I always kept a half dozen extra containers just in case. (I went through it so eventually I prepared for it.)

You still need to figure out timing and meal plans but we will get to that.

Planning Your Workouts

You should plan for two workouts per day, six days a week. That covers both cardio and regular workouts. The routine that I liked the best was working out 3 days per week, Monday, Wednesday and Friday of major muscle groups, and using Saturday to do the smaller muscles that didn't always get hit so hard, like traps or calves. Also, plan on doing cardio every morning for a half hour minimum. Just be aware at this point that you will need basically an hour and a half, twice a day, for six days a week. One day of complete rest is really needed when you're going at this level, so take one day off.

In my own program, I did my cardio from 5 until 5:30 or 6 every morning. Every afternoon when I got off work I hit the gym again from about 4 until 5:30 in the afternoon.

There are adjustments that have to be made as you go depending on whether you are in a building phase or a cutting phase. (Packing on muscle or stripping off fat.)

Building and Cutting

As you go through your program, you will need to coordinate your diet and exercise/cardio in "cycles" to give yourself the optimum benefit of building muscle but also stripping off body fat. The best way this is done, is by cycling your workouts. Typically, you would have a 7-10 day period where you consume more calories and focus more on actual workouts with weights or resistance exercises to build muscle. During this time, you would also adjust your supplement intake to preserve and foster muscle growth. Then, in your next 7-10 day cycle, you would decrease calorie intake and focus your workout more on intense fat burning cardio. By doing it this way, you get the best of both.

During both the building and the cutting phase, you would be doing both weight training and cardio. The difference comes in the amount that you do. The diet part during these phases is a bit more precise because in getting ripped, the kinds and amounts of calories you consume is a huge key.

Preparation Summary

I have given you an overview of the things that you will be looking at or focusing on during your transformation period. Workouts, cardio, diet, attitude, focus, supplements, timing, intensity and other factors will all come into play for your transformation. Each person is different and there will be minor adjustments to the program I am about to lay out. Things like food preferences and amounts you may have to adjust slightly, but the concept of the way to get ripped in a short amount of time is right on. Please really give serious thought to the things I have told you and to the things I am about to tell you.

Also know this going in... There are going to be people who will disagree with all this. You will have people who are huge and muscular who will tell you that you need to do this or that differently. The temptation is to think, "Look at them! They are built! They must know what they are talking about." And when it comes to training and workouts in general, they probably do. But to get ripped is a different thing, especially if you are doing a contest. At the end of 12 weeks or however many weeks the contest is, you will see that the photos don't lie. Take the photo of the built guy and put it next to the photo of the ripped guy and I can tell you who will win. It doesn't even matter at that point that the built guy's arms are two inches bigger or his shoulders a little wider. You can't tell any of that stuff by looking at the photo. Losing that extra quarter inch of body fat makes all the difference in the world.

These things are the difference between doing a "decent job" of your transformation and doing what it really takes to get the job done. Period.

3
THE BREAKDOWN

In this section, I'm going to be real specific about my own program. Keep in mind that your exercises and calories etc., will vary slightly according to what your body is telling you. (for instance.. I dropped down to a body weight that was too low for me and I lost strength to the point where I felt weak a lot. My body was telling me to put those five lbs. back on.)

The Workout

Keep in mind here that we are not re-inventing the wheel. This is not the time to search out weird new exercises, or for trying things that may, or may not, be helpful. Stick with what you know. The basics will be perfect for our purposes.

Body parts
We are going to be focusing on these muscle "groups." Back, chest, biceps, triceps, shoulders, traps, abdominals, quadriceps, hamstrings and calves. Of course there are other muscles that are important that will be "hit" or affected when you do the exercise for the major muscle. Such as glutes will receive a workout during the leg workout naturally.

Back – Traps, Lats, Middle Back and Lower back

Body part - Traps

Shrugs-Dumbbell...*Using a weight that is moderately challenging but not ridiculous, stand with feet about shoulder width and hold dumbbells at your side. While keeping your arms reasonably strait, slowly raise your shoulders up to your ears as if "shrugging." Focus your attention on the muscle and feel it work. Make every rep count.

3 sets x 10 reps per set

*I had started out using 20 lbs. for curls and using 30 lbs. for shrugs. I increased it eventually to 50 lbs. as I was able to do so.

Shrugs-Barbell ... (shoulder width grip) Again, standing with feet at shoulder width, grasp barbell with a shoulder width grip and stand strait. Slowly lift bar up by shrugging your shoulders so that your shoulders are drawn up close to your ears. Make each rep count.

3 sets x 8 reps per set

Close grip shrug/upright row... This exercise also hits your shoulders as well. Standing with feet at shoulder width, grasp barbell with hands together or fairly close together (overhand) and lift bar up towards your chin. Also pay attention to do a similar motion as you did for the shrugs and focus on your traps.

3 sets x 8 reps per set

Body part , Lats, Middle and Lower Back

Seated low cable rows... As you pull back, don't lean back but come to an upright seated position. Continue to move the weight by pulling your elbows back and constricting your back muscles as you pull back. Don't allow your lower back to do the work. When you go forward in the movement, allow yourself to stretch out and get a nice stretch. Your body will thank you. * You should be able to handle a fairly heavy weight because of the strength of your back naturally. Always choose a weight that challenges you, but you shouldn't choose a weight so heavy that you can't easily complete your full 3 sets x 8 to 10 reps. You can always give the exercise more focus to increase the resistance.

3 sets x 10 reps per set

Dumbbell rows... This was one of my favorite back exercises because the freedom of movement really lets you squeeze the muscle at the top of the movement. Your focus is also better because you are hitting only one side at a time. Using a freestanding bench press bench, place your knee on the bench and also your hand of the same side and lean over to do a bent over row. (left knee/left hand etc.) using the opposite hand, hold the dumbbell. So placing your body in a horizontal position, draw the weight up to where the dumbbell comes close to, or alongside of your chest. When you get to the top of the movement, make sure to squeeze, contracting the muscle just a little bit more.

3 sets x 8 reps per set (both sides)

Lat Pulldowns... I like the simplicity of this exercise and the effectiveness. Choose a weight that will allow you to put more effort into it than is required. Also in this exercise, squeeze a little more at the top of the movement. I like to alternate sets of behind the neck and in front. (i.e. one set behind...next set in front)

4 sets x 8 reps per set (2 in front and 2 behind)
Bent Over Barbell Rows...Because the back is typically such a strong and powerful set of muscles, sometimes you have to challenge yourself to go that little extra that causes muscle growth. On this particular exercise, I do this at the end of my back workout or

sometimes at the end of my workout, depending on how hard I want to hit the smaller muscle groups. This is a burnout set. Using a fairly light weight, do reps to failure (where you can't do anymore in good form) This is just a finisher to get a good pump in your back muscles.

1 set to failure

Body part – Chest

Machine bench press... Unless you have a committed training partner to do free weights with, I suggest using the machines. You are not dependent on someone to show up to start your workout and you can safely use heavy weights that focus on the major muscles. The supporting muscles still get a bit of the workout but with free weights your supporting muscles play a bigger role to stabilize the weight therefor you can't go as heavy as you might have otherwise. This is really true if you are working out alone.

Use a weight that is heavy enough that you have to work to get 10 reps... but do only 8. (so you can purposely put extra effort through focus.)

4 sets x 8 reps

Dumbbell bench press... I love this one also. You can really get a good workout with this exercise. As in our other exercises, choose a weight that is about 80% of your max ability. As you sit on the end of the bench, hold the dumbbells on your thighs and then lay back on the bench while bringing the dumbbells onto your chest. I like to start with the dumbbell in a position where they are perpendicular to your body. In other words, your hand position is like it would be if you were carrying a suitcase. At the top of the movement, rotate your hands slightly where your thumbs are facing together and bring the dumbbells together lightly while squeezing your pecs together.

On this particular exercise, I don't recommend dipping the weights much lower than the level of your chest. (maybe slightly) Using heavy weights and doing that is a good way to sustain shoulder injuries if you are not already in excellent shape.

At the end of each set, just let the weights softly drop to the floor.

3 to 4 sets x 8 reps

Pec Deck… Another great exercise for getting a good "pump." This machine is designed so that you naturally squeeze your chest muscles together at the top of the movement. In doing this exercise, don't let the machine go all the way back to starting position unless you need to rest. Keep a little tension on the muscles as you work them. Use a weight that challenges you but save enough of yourself that you can really give your chest a nice "squeeze" at the top of the movement.

4 sets x 8 reps

Body part – Shoulders

Dumbbell shoulder press... From a seated position press the dumbbells upwards bringing them together slightly at the top of the movement. In my opinion, this is the core exercise for shoulders. Use a slightly lighter weight than you need to, making up for it by doing extra reps.

4 sets x 10 reps

Bent-over rear-delt raise (flys)... From a standing, slightly bent over position, move the dumbbells in a motion away from your body while lifting your arms as if you are spreading your wings. (hence... flys) Again, don't use extremely heavy weights for this exercise but only slightly challenging. Especially for muscle groups such as shoulders, get your pump from the extra focus not the extra weight. It will keep you from being sidelined buy injury. The tendency sometimes is to get a momentum going as if you really are trying to fly, but I like a more controlled pace where you focus on the muscle and the movement.

3 sets x 8 reps

Dumbbell lateral raise... From a standing position holding the dumbbells at your side, lift them up to the side away from your body while keeping your arms fairly strait. This exercise was more of a finisher for me. Even though I was able to use much more weight, I used 10 or 15 lb. dumbbells.

3 sets x 8 reps

Body Part – Biceps

E-Z curl bar curls...Start your biceps workout using the bar and the slightly heavier weight. I prefer the E-z curl bar but you can also use the strait Olympic bar if you find it easier or more effective for you. From a standing position, I like doing this movement semi-slow, focusing hard on the muscle and how it feels. Contract the biceps hard at the top of the movement. Don't use a weight that challenges your joints...just your muscles.

4 sets x 8 reps

Seated alternate dumbbell curls... You can do this exercise with either a strait back chair or use one that is slightly leaning back. I always preferred the one that leans back. From your seated position, let the weights hang at your sides. Draw up one dumbbell at a time, alternating the reps. Let the transition between left and right reps be smooth and controlled, remembering to squeeze at the top of the movement slightly.

4 sets x 8 reps

Concentration curls... This is where you are seated with the arm that is doing the reps placed between your legs with your elbow rested on your inner thigh. You use your thigh as a base or platform from which to do the curl. This is one exercise where concentration on the muscle and movement is what defines the exercise. Alternate arms by doing 1 set left and then 1 set right etc..

3 sets x 8 reps (each side)

Burnout dumbbell curls... A great way to finish a biceps workout. Starting with the weight that you normally do curls with, do 10-12 reps and then move immediately to the next lowest weight (no rest between sets) and do 10-12 reps and so on until you finish by using 10s.
6 sets (approx.) x 40,35,30,25,20 & 15 lbs. (for example)

Body part- Triceps

Cable push-down... While placing your elbows close to your body, and your hands close together on the small bar, push the bar down in a controlled and concentrated motion. Again, squeezing at the top of the movement. Typically you should be able to do a decent amount of weight with this exercise. Because this is a machine exercise, this is the one that we do the heavier weight.

4 sets x 8 to 10 reps

Mule kicks... This exercise starts out similar to the dumbbell row. You are kneeling with one knee on the bench, also supporting yourself with one hand on the bench. Instead of drawing the weight up in a "row", you push the weight up and back behind you like a mule would kick. I like to use a lighter weight for these, focusing on the movement.

4 sets x 8 reps

Seated Overhead Dumbbell Extension...Use a seat with a back to give you added stability for this one. Using the arm you are starting with, lift the weight above your head. Then take your other arm and reach behind your head to stabilize your other arm by grabbing hold of your arm. (i.e. You are doing reps with your right, so you reach behind your head with your left, holding your right biceps with your left hand)

Then slowly lower the weight behind your head while keeping your elbow pointed toward the ceiling, then push the weight back up. This is also a great exercise for building mass for the long triceps head.

3 to 4 sets x 8 reps

Body part – Quadriceps & Hamstrings (& Glutes)

Leg extensions... Using the leg extension machine, set your weight where you are barely getting through the 8 reps of your set. Legs because of constant use recover fairly quickly so you can work them harder than the other body parts. Also something good to keep in mind is the fact that because the leg muscle are so large, they burn a lot of calories for you. (Making fat loss easier.) So give them a good workout!

4 sets x 8 reps

Hamstring curls... I love this exercise but it sure feels strange. You do it on a hamstring curl machine. It is not a natural movement that your leg would make with resistance, so it may feel a bit strange when you do it. (in a good way) Again use a weight that will allow you to squeeze the muscle at the top of the rep.

4 sets x 8 reps

Leg press...Use as heavy as you are able to while still maintaining control and good form. Do four sets while increasing the weight as your legs "warm up." You can experiment with foot positions if you like. I would point my toes strait up for one set and then facing out for one set and the facing in for the next. Then I would finish with them back at the original position.

4 sets x 8 reps (example 1 set at 250lbs., then increase to 300 etc..)

Walking lunges (Grouchos)... These were some of my favorite leg exercises. You can really feel these. These are basically lunges where instead of going back to your original starting position, you take another "step." Do 10 steps per set. As you lunge, do not let your knee touch the ground but just come close to it. After you get use to the movement, do these lunges while carrying dumbbells in each hand. As heavy as you can while maintaining control.

4 sets x 10 steps

Body part – Calves

Calf raise... For calves, there really is not an abundance of different exercises that you can do. Calf raises do the trick if you use a little weight and focus on the movement. I always did more reps for calves and it worked well.

5-6 sets x 15 reps

You can also do your calves on the leg press if you prefer by placing your toes on the edge of the plate. Either in addition to or in place of...

Body part – Abdominals

The misunderstanding about having great abs is so wide-spread. For years I used to think if you just did the right ab workout, you could have those abs like we see in the magazines. Oh the wasted years! Yes, you do need some good ab exercises. That part is true. You have to have some nice muscles beneath the fat once it is stripped away. But the real key to those abs we will get to in a bit. First let's talk exercise... Although you may eventually fine tune your exercises to hit and develop all the little muscles that give you a more perfectly sculpted physique, you can get your abs with three great moves...

Crunch # 1... Lay on your back with your legs bent and resting over or on a workout bench. While holding your arms and hands in front of you (Maybe crossed upon your chest) and not behind your head, do a partial sit up (crunch) and hold that crunch for 3 to 4 seconds. Really focus on the movement and the muscle.

3 sets of 20 crunches

Crunch #2... While laying on the floor on your back, reach above your head and hold onto a bench or stable apparatus of some sort to stabilize yourself. Then lift your legs off the ground a couple of inches in a short-lived leg raise, drawing your knees up to your chest. Hold that crunched position several seconds and repeat.

3 sets of 20 crunches

Crunch #3... The twisting crunch. Lay on the floor and place your hands near the sides of your head. (again, not behind your head) in a combination movement of part sit up, twist and leg lift, lift your left knee and your right elbow towards each other, then repeat the movement with your right knee and left elbow. Don't rest between reps. Do this continually for 20 times before resting. Always make each rep count.

3 sets of 20 crunches

Exercise Overview

I know these exercises that I have laid out seem very basic and easy and not at all complicated. It really doesn't even seem as if I've given you enough to do does it? Keep in mind that these muscle groups will be spread out over a week and then it really seems like it's not enough. But it is. You have to understand that because of the calorie restrictions you will not have the fuel to keep exercising endlessly without tearing down muscle and not allowing it to repair. You have to give it all you have for that hour and a half and get the job done in that time frame. Because you will still need some of that energy for the cardio. It's a package deal. Every piece is important to pack on muscle and get ripped at the same time. It's a balance.

Cardio

I mentioned in the beginning my understanding of cardio, and how one would best benefit from it. From all the literature I had read, I never really understood just how important and critical this part of the equation was. After 2 seriously flawed attempts at getting ripped for the transformation challenge, I started doing more searching instead of the surface stuff I had been reading in the fitness magazines.

One thing that really stood out to me was this. Competitive bodybuilders will do up to 2 hours of cardio a day to get ready for a contest. Two hours! And they are already in really good shape! As I investigated this, I saw that this was the norm. This wasn't the exception. In my second attempt I had done more cardio but going into my third try, I reevaluated my cardio altogether.

Here was what I came up with... On days when I was not working out, I did and hour and a half of intensive cardio. On the days I was working out, I did forty-five minutes to an hour. No coasting, just hardcore cardio. Here was how it played out.

I will mention some alternatives, but for the most part my cardio was done on a recumbent bike. I found that I could expend the most energy but not lose momentum if I had to coast for a minute to catch my breath. If you are on a treadmill or a stair-stepper and you stop to catch your breath, you are stopped. On a bike you can set the level to nothing and keep moving your legs while you catch your breath and get a drink.

So, I get my water bottle and 2 towels for my cardio workout. One towel is a small one to wipe my face with. The other towel is a large towel to fold up and sit on to absorb the sweat from my workout. I'm telling you these details so that you can see that the workout is intense enough that I need a large towel. I keep the water bottle handy and take a drink about every 3 to 5 minutes.

I start on the bike and do a two -minute warmup on a low resistance setting. After my initial warmup, I increase the difficulty level by one, every minute until I am at the maximum level. I am not slogging through this. I am "sprinting" so to speak as I go. After a few minutes I am breathing hard and I settle into a "routine" of rhythmic deep breaths so that I can continue this pace. I would go for 30 minutes and according to the meter on the bike I would burn about 750 calories.

At this point, I would get up and go refill my water bottle, walk around the gym for five minutes and catch my breath. Then I would do it again. Even though it was only one hour of cardio, by the time I was done, I had burned

1,500 calories and was completely soaked... my socks, my underwear, everything. I didn't understand just how effective this cardio thing was until I weighed myself one day. One that particular day I weighed 211 lbs. when I arrived at the gym. After one hour of cardio I weighed 206. I realize that it was mostly water weight but that told me something. If you are trying to lose the last few lbs. of water weight before taking an after picture, this would be one very effective way to do it.

To be completely transparent with you, my morning cardio was not quite that intense. I still worked up a sweat but my clothes were only damp and I only needed one towel. I was riding my own exercise bike in the mornings at home. I would get up, drink 2 big glasses of water and then jump on the bike. I don't think that I was awake enough to be too extreme. But it jump started my metabolism for the day.

The Exercise Bike... I've already given you the description but I prefer the recumbent bikes. After initial warmup take it to the highest level that you can maintain and push yourself to go for more.

6 Days per Week / split routine / workout days... 45 min. to an hour / non workout days...30-45 minutes in the morning and 2- 30 minute sessions back to back in the afternoon.

The Stair-stepper... Also a great cardio workout. The first time I got on it at the beginning of my program, I pushed myself to do six minutes. I thought I would die. You can do the same cardio program with the stair stepper if you prefer or mix and match. As I said I prefer the bike because I don't like to lose momentum if I need to catch my breath.

The Treadmill... Although I did use it a few times, it did not lend itself to accomplishing what I needed. You would have to run full out and on a treadmill it's not easy to do. It would be better to run outside on a track if you prefer to run.

4
FOOD AND SUPPLEMENTS

The Food Intake

This is also a very important aspect of the transformation. Not having good advice really messed me up the first couple of times. I started out weighing 250 lbs. I needed to lose about 50 lbs. By all conventional wisdom in the magazines I was reading at the time, I should have been consuming 3,500 calories per day. (6 meals times 600 calories)

The articles were very compelling on why you have to eat that much. They talked about lean this and low fat that and how eating these certain foods kept the metabolism going etc.. In the end, it just didn't work for me. I had to lose 50 lbs. of fat and consuming 3,500 calories per day just did not get the job done.

For my third go around, these were my numbers... On my building phase my calorie intake was 1,800 to 2,000 calories per day split into 6 meals. On my cutting phase my calories were about 1,500 per day also split up into 6 meals. This amount of calories gave me sufficient energy to do my workouts the way I have laid them out and still build muscle and lose fat. The numbers worked. The key to not being hungry is getting used to the amount (took a couple of weeks) and finding no or low calorie foods that will fill you up. For instance, green beans is considered to be a "negative" food. That means that although a can of green beans has 70 calories, your body has to expend more calories than that to digest and process it. Therefor its a negative food.

So... Now that you have a more realistic idea of calorie intake to win a transformation contest let's look at some foods.

The kind of foods that you need are proteins, fibrous carbs, complex carbs and fats.

Proteins

Tuna fish... 6 oz. can is about 160 – 190 calories of almost pure protein.
Chicken...   6 oz. of chicken breast is about 275 calories.
Lean beef... 6 oz. of Lean beef is about 550 calories.
**This tells me right away that my "real food"

protein for the next 12 weeks is going to be tuna. When I read in the food intake info about getting ripped for contests it talked about the importance of eating different foods to have a little variety and not get burned out etc.. No, we can have variety after the 12 weeks are over. For now, we are just going to focus on success and not whether or not we feel deprived of variety.

** We can also get our protein from protein powders.

Complex Carbs

Complex carbs are important to keep your blood sugar level and provide consistent energy throughout the day for living in general and for our workouts.

Oatmeal... ½ cup is about 150 calories
Brown Rice (Long grain) 1 cup is about 210 calories
Whole Wheat Pasta ...1 cup is about 170 calories
Black Beans... 1 cup is about 220 calories
Sweet Potato...1 cup is about 110 calories
I could go through a long list of foods that I checked out while trying to come up with the best foods for my purpose. Although there are lots of foods recommended for getting in shape or getting healthy, in the end I had to choose the things that would help me accomplish my goals... In the end, oatmeal was my carb of

choice with sweet potato 2 or 3 times per week. Occasionally I would also eat brown rice or pasta but that was pretty much it.

Fibrous Carbs

Green Beans... 1 cup is about 30 calories (1 can is about 70 calories)
Broccoli ...1 cup is about 30 calories
Lettuce... 1 cup is about 5 calories
The trick is to find high fiber vegetables that you like that are also low in calorie. These were mine. There were many more that I could have chosen but I had to take into consideration that I had already done the transformation competition twice so I was not so much looking to be comfortable as successful.

No Calorie Foods

Dill Pickle... about 20 calories
Medium sized tomato... about 25 calories
2 Large Celery Stalks... about 12 calories
½ Cucumber...about 20 calories
These are a few of the very low calorie foods. They are handy to have on hand, just in case you get hungry.
I preferred dill pickles. However there are several more that you can probably find online.

My Meals

My meals during the building phase were effective but not full of variety. I was doing 300 calories per meal, six meals per day. They looked very similar to this

Meal 1 – ½ cup of oatmeal 150 cal. Mixed with ½ packet protein powder 145 cal.

Meal 2 – ½ cup oatmeal / ½ pack protein powder / ½ tsp natural peanut butter

Meal 3 – 1 sm. Sweet potato 125 cal. And 1 can of tuna 160 cal.

Meal 4 – (pre-workout meal) 1 meal replacement shake 280 calories

Meal 5 – (post- workout) 1 meal replacement shake w/ simple sugar creatine 100 cal.

Meal 6 – ½ cup oatmeal or 1 cup pasta (150 cal.) tuna or protein powder.

During this phase, I tried to eat just slightly more carbs to fuel my workouts. I rotated these few different foods in and out, just mindful of the calorie intake. The days when I was really hungry I would snack on the super low calorie foods.

During the cutting phase my meals were even more restricted in their lack of variety. My calorie intake was about 250 per meal.

Meal 1 – 1 can tuna 160 cal. and 1 can or cup green beans 70 cal.

Meal 2 – 1 can tuna and 1 can green beans

Meal 3 – 1 small chicken breast 200-250 cal. 1 cup broccoli 30 cal.

Meal 4 – 1 meal replacement shake

Meal 5 – 1 meal replacement shake w/ simple sugar glutamine

Meal 6 – 1 can tuna and 1 can green beans or 200 calories worth of protein powder.

Again I mixed and matched to give myself a little bit of change and kept the dill pickles and celery handy especially during the cutting phase because it seems like you can be a lot hungrier during this phase.

It was really not a great sacrifice to change the way I ate during this contest. The hardest part was being around people who expect you to eat.

Supplements

I used only a few different things during the third competition. I had used metabolism enhancers during the first contest but I did not feel that it really helped me.

1 Meal Replacements – For my pre and post workout meals I tried to use these meals because they were already broken down. I felt it was easier for my body to have what it needed

faster to help fuel the workout and to replenish itself post workout.

2 Protein Powder – Having so few protein choices I felt that this processed protein would give me the option of protein to mix with my oatmeal and also protein as dessert. A little protein powder mixed with cold water is kind of like a healthy pudding.

3 Creatine (creatinine) - Helps foster muscle growth. I would use this exclusively during my building phase, but definitely not when cutting or getting ready for pictures. It causes your muscles to retain water, giving a smooth somewhat bloated look.

4 Glutamine – a supplement that reduces muscle catabolism and breakdown of muscle during stress. It keeps your muscle intact during your workouts on restricted calorie intake. Use this especially during cutting phases.

** Initially I had used a few other products offered by the company because they were recommended. (And I thought that using more of the products would give me a better chance.) But in the end, the four things that I listed above were all I needed.

The Cheat Day

This is a popular concept in the bodybuilding / workout world. A day where you do off of your diet to keep your sanity so to speak. It does make sense to give yourself one day a week so that you don't feel tempted all of the time to go off your clean eating program. The problem is that when you are doing a contest where you only have so much time to reach your goal, you can't have a cheat day. You have to pare it down to only a cheat meal. I know this firsthand because during my first two competitions, I fully took advantage of the cheat day concept. After all, the sponsoring company suggested it! I realized at a point too late that it was derailing my success and I stopped.

Take advantage of a cheat meal once a week. But do not let it get out of hand. Eat an entire pizza after the competition, not during the competition! During my third go-round, I ate about 600-700 calories for my cheat meal. My body seemed to be able to handle that and it created no issue whatsoever. I did have one cheat meal where I ate about 2,000 calories and I think because it was an isolated incident, it also did not create a problem.
My advice is yes, do the cheat deal but not the cheat day

The Mental Reinforcement

I mentioned earlier about having some kind of mental image about what you want your success to look like. In my own case, I took several, really great photos from a popular health magazine and put them in a folder where I could take a glance at them throughout my day. I would spend just a few minutes "seeing" myself with the physique that those on the pictures had. It was a great reinforcement. I suggest that you do the same. (I am also writing a more "in depth" explanation on this aspect of positive reinforcement. I will offer it as well at low or no cost to those who would like to know more about it.)

5
PUTTING IT TOGETHER

Now you have pretty much all of the pieces that I believe you need to have to be successful and win a transformation challenge. The only other thing that makes a difference at this point is your desire and level of commitment.

Here is an overview of my workouts

The way I had my workouts laid out, I was working each body part once a week. Of course, you know that anytime you work one area, the other areas have to support your workout as well. The other areas will get "hit" residually from each workout. But you still have to make each workout really count because of this. During your hour and a half workout, you have to be all in, just like for the cardio portion. No coasting for that hour if you can help it. There is time to relax afterwards.

I did 2 muscle groups per workout for the most part, with the smaller groups getting hit on cardio days. It looked like this....

Sunday – off

Monday – A.M. Cardio 30-45 min. / Back and Biceps workout

Tuesday – A.M. Cardio 45 min. / Ab workout / P.M. Cardio 2- 30 min. sessions

Wednesday – A.M. Cardio 30-45 min. / Legs workout / no P.M. Cardio

Thursday – A.M. Cardio 45 min. / Ab workout / P.M. Cardio 2-30 min. sessions

Friday – A.M. Cardio 30-45 min. / Chest and Triceps workout

Saturday – A.M. Cardio 45 min. / Shoulder workout plus any body part that I felt did not get hit hard enough in my weekly workout. (calves) / P.M. Cardio 2-30 min. sessions

**This was the schedule during my building phase. During the cutting phase, I added P.M. Cardio after my workouts as well.

It doesn't look like much, but if you are focused it can be what you need. As I mentioned, you will be restricting your calories so your workout cannot go on forever if you want to see growth.

The exercises that I used are the exact ones that I listed earlier. Each exercise and set and rep is what I have told you about.

Phases or Cycles

Over my 12 week period I found it best to cycle my building and cutting time periods at between 7-10 days each. So I would do my building phase for 10 days, eating additional calories, doing less cardio and supplementing with creatine.

Then I would do my cutting phase where my calories were more restricted, I increased my cardio by adding P.M. cardio after my workouts and I supplemented with glutamine.

If you begin to feel weak, you can add additional calories (carbs) to give you strength as long as they are healthy carbs and not simple sugar carbs.

Success in Transformation !

The overall concept and plan that I have presented to you is kind of a flip-flop of the current wisdom on this subject. That is why this is the successful approach. In the past, it was all about the workout. Spending hours in the gym, trying to get bigger and more muscular, eating lots of good calories and moderating your cardio so as not to break down your muscle. I have seen a lot of people who take this approach.

This recipe is showing that all of the parts are important. Focus and dedication and passion play a huge role. You can do this! Whether you are competing in a competition or just getting ready for summer, you can do this!

Conclusion

I was doing seated dumbbell presses one afternoon at the gym. I had been on attempt number three for about 9 weeks or so. I was watching the muscles in my arms separate and move as I lifted the weight and lowered it. I will be honest and tell you that at that point I was really proud of this accomplishment. I had never seen my body looking like that. As I finished my set, and was getting up from the bench, one of the young trainers at the gym came over to me. I had not talked to him before but he introduced himself and told me "I've been watching you work out. I just had to come and tell you that you are one of the best built guys in this gym." He shook my hand and walked away.

Only a couple months earlier I had been overweight and out of shape...

You can do this...

About the Author

Michael Smyth is a writer with a desire to show people that through simple but effective strategies, they can literally mold their bodies into something to be proud of and be in the best shape of their lives.

GETTING RIPPED